STAYING FIT AND HEALTHY DURING PREGNANCY

A Complete Guide-to Exercise for First Time Moms and Cookbook to Help Them with Nutrition

Danny Graham

Disclaimer

The information provided in this guide and cookbook is for general guidance and educational purposes only. It is not a substitute for professional medical advice, diagnosis, or treatment. Always consult with your healthcare provider before starting any exercise program or making significant dietary changes, especially during pregnancy or postpartum. The authors and publishers disclaim any liability for any adverse effects or consequences resulting from the use of the information herein. Every individual's health circumstances are unique; personalized advice from qualified professionals is recommended. Readers are encouraged to use their discretion and seek appropriate guidance for their specific situations.

Contents

CHAPTER 1

The Exciting Beginning

1.1 Embracing Motherhood and Fitness

The journey into motherhood is an exhilarating and transformative experience, marked by the anticipation of new life and the profound changes happening within. Amidst the excitement, it is crucial for expectant mothers to embrace a holistic approach to well-being, where the integration of motherhood and fitness plays a pivotal role.

1.1.1 The Symbiosis of Motherhood and Fitness

The intersection of motherhood and fitness is not only compatible but also mutually reinforcing. Engaging in regular, moderate exercise during pregnancy has been shown to have a multitude of benefits for both the mother and the developing baby. From improved cardiovascular health to better mood regulation, the positive impacts of staying active are numerous.

Explore the various forms of exercise suitable for expectant mothers, ranging from low-impact aerobics activities to specialized prenatal yoga. Understand how these exercises can enhance muscular strength, flexibility, and overall endurance, preparing the body for the physical demands of pregnancy and childbirth.

1.1.2 Navigating Safety and Adaptations

While embracing fitness during pregnancy is encouraged, safety considerations are paramount. Delve into detailed guidelines on exercising safely during each trimester, understanding the body's changing needs and limitations. Learn about suitable modifications and adaptations for different fitness routines, ensuring a comfortable and risk-free experience.

Address common concerns and myths surrounding exercise during pregnancy, empowering mothers-to-be with evidence-based information. By understanding the intricacies of maintaining a fitness routine while pregnant, expectant mothers can confidently embrace a healthy, active lifestyle.

1.1.3 The Mental and Emotional Benefits

Beyond the physical advantages, the mental and emotional benefits of incorporating fitness into pregnancy are profound. Explore how regular exercise can alleviate stress, anxiety, and mood swings, contributing to a more positive and balanced emotional state. Delve into the connection between physical activity and improved sleep quality, a crucial aspect of well-being during pregnancy.

Discover the community aspect of prenatal fitness classes and support groups, fostering connections with other expectant mothers. The shared experiences in these settings not only create a sense of camaraderie but also provide a platform for valuable information exchange.

1.1.4 Embracing Body Positivity and Self-Care

As the body undergoes remarkable changes, embracing body positivity becomes a cornerstone of the motherhood and fitness journey. Explore strategies for cultivating a positive body image, understanding that each pregnancy is unique, and every woman's experience is different. Dive into the concept of self-care, recognizing the importance of rest, relaxation, and mindfulness in promoting overall well-being.

Celebrate the beauty of the changing body and explore self-care practices that nurture both the physical and emotional aspects of the mother-to-be. By embracing a positive mindset and fostering self-love, expectant mothers can navigate the transformative journey of pregnancy with confidence and grace.

1.2 Navigating the Unique Challenges of First-Time Moms

The excitement of becoming a mother for the first time is unparalleled, but it also brings forth a set of unique challenges and uncertainties. From the initial discovery of pregnancy to the postpartum period, first-time moms navigate uncharted territory, seeking guidance and understanding. This section provides insights into the distinctive challenges faced by first-time mothers and offers practical tips for a smoother transition into motherhood.

1.2.1 Preparing for the Unknown

The journey of a first-time mom begins with the revelation of pregnancy, a moment filled with joy and perhaps a touch of apprehension. Delve into the emotions and concerns that often accompany this revelation, exploring strategies for preparing mentally and emotionally for the unknown.

Understand the importance of seeking prenatal care early in the pregnancy journey and establishing a strong support network. Learn from the experiences of seasoned mothers, gaining insights into the realities of pregnancy and childbirth that may not be readily apparent.

1.2.2 Anticipating the Unpredictable

The path to motherhood is seldom a linear one, and first-time moms often find themselves facing unexpected challenges. Explore common surprises and uncertainties that can arise during pregnancy, childbirth, and the postpartum period. From unexpected changes in birth plans to the emotional rollercoaster of postpartum adjustment, gain a comprehensive understanding of what lies ahead.

Navigate the unpredictable aspects of motherhood with resilience and adaptability. Learn how to embrace flexibility in expectations, empowering yourself to face challenges with a proactive and positive mindset.

1.2.3 Building a Supportive Network

The importance of a supportive network cannot be overstated for first-time mothers. Dive into strategies for building a strong support system, encompassing partners, family, friends, and healthcare professionals. Understand the significance of open communication and the role of emotional support in navigating the challenges of motherhood.

Explore the dynamics of partner involvement during pregnancy and childbirth, fostering a sense of shared responsibility and connection. Learn from the experiences of other first-time moms, gaining insights into the various ways a support network can make a significant difference in the journey into motherhood.

1.2.4 Postpartum Realities and Self-Care

The postpartum period brings its own set of challenges, often catching first-time moms off guard. Delve into the physical and emotional changes that accompany the postpartum phase, exploring self-care practices that promote healing and well-being. From managing sleep deprivation to addressing postpartum blues, gain insights into the realities of the postpartum experience.

Understand the importance of seeking professional help when needed, recognizing that postpartum mental health is a critical aspect of overall well-being. By acknowledging the challenges and embracing self-care strategies, first-time moms can navigate the postpartum period with resilience and self-compassion.

1.3 Setting Goals for a Healthy Pregnancy

A healthy pregnancy is a multifaceted journey that goes beyond routine medical check-ups. Setting intentional and realistic goals is a proactive approach that empowers expectant mothers to prioritize their well-being and that of their growing baby. This section explores the various dimensions of goal-setting for a healthy pregnancy, encompassing nutrition, fitness, mental health, and overall wellness.

1.3.1 Nourishing the Body for Two

Nutrition forms the foundation of a healthy pregnancy, influencing the development of the baby and the well-being of the mother. Dive into the intricacies of prenatal nutrition, exploring the essential nutrients needed during each trimester. From the importance of folic acid to the role of omega-3 fatty acids, gain insights into creating a balanced and nourishing diet.

Explore strategies for managing common pregnancy-related discomforts through nutrition, from morning sickness to gestational diabetes. Understand the concept of mindful eating and intuitive nutrition, fostering a positive relationship with food during this transformative phase.

1.3.2 Tailoring Fitness Goals to Pregnancy

Setting fitness goals during pregnancy involves a thoughtful and adaptive approach. Delve into the benefits of maintaining physical activity throughout pregnancy, understanding the role of exercise in promoting overall health. Explore suitable exercises for different stages of pregnancy, from gentle prenatal yoga to low-impact cardiovascular activities.

Understand the importance of listening to the body, making necessary modifications to fitness routines, and embracing a variety of exercises that contribute to strength, flexibility, and cardiovascular fitness. By setting realistic fitness goals, expectant mothers can enhance their physical well-being and prepare their bodies for the demands of childbirth.

1.3.3 Prioritizing Mental Health and Emotional Well-Being

The mental and emotional well-being of an expectant mother is intricately connected to the health of the pregnancy. Explore strategies for managing stress, anxiety, and mood swings during pregnancy, fostering a positive and resilient mindset. Understand the role of relaxation techniques, mindfulness, and emotional support in promoting mental health.

Delve into the concept of setting realistic expectations for oneself and cultivating a positive self-image. Recognize the importance of seeking professional help when needed, understanding that mental health is an integral component of a healthy pregnancy.

1.3.4 Embracing Holistic Wellness

A healthy pregnancy extends beyond physical and mental well-being, encompassing holistic wellness. Explore practices that contribute to overall wellness, from adequate sleep to hydration and stress management. Understand the importance of regular prenatal check-ups, monitoring the baby's development, and addressing any concerns promptly.

Dive into the concept of birth planning, where expectant mothers can set intentions and preferences for their childbirth experience. Explore the various birthing options available and gain insights into creating a supportive birthing environment that aligns with personal preferences and values.

1.3.5 Fostering a Positive Birth Experience

Setting goals for a healthy pregnancy includes considerations for the birth experience itself. Explore childbirth education, birthing plans, and the role of informed decision-making in shaping a positive birth experience. Understand the various birthing options available, from natural childbirth to medical interventions, and make decisions that align with personal preferences.

Explore the importance of open communication with healthcare providers, creating a collaborative and supportive birthing team. By setting goals for a positive birth experience, expectant mothers can approach childbirth with confidence, knowledge, and a sense of empowerment.

holistic well-being.

CHAPTER 2

Understanding Your Changing Body

2.1 Physiological Changes During Pregnancy

The miracle of pregnancy brings about a myriad of physiological changes within a woman's body, each contributing to the nurturing and development of the growing baby. Understanding these changes is not only crucial for expectant mothers but also empowers them to embrace the transformative journey with knowledge and self-awareness.

2.1.1 The Marvel of Conception and Early Changes

The journey of pregnancy begins with the miracle of conception, where a fertilized egg implants itself into the uterine lining. Delve into the early physiological changes that mark the beginning of pregnancy, from the formation of the placenta to the initiation of hormonal shifts. Understand the role of hormones such as human chorionic gonadotropin (HCG) and progesterone in supporting and sustaining early pregnancy.

Explore the concept of embryonic development, tracing the formation of vital organs and the establishment of the amniotic sac. Gain insights into the early symptoms of pregnancy, from morning sickness to changes in breast size and sensitivity.

2.1.2 Cardiovascular and Respiratory Adaptations

As pregnancy progresses, the cardiovascular and respiratory systems undergo significant adaptations to meet the increasing demands of both the mother and the developing baby. Delve into the changes in blood volume, heart rate, and cardiac output, understanding how these adjustments contribute to the circulatory needs of pregnancy.

Explore the impact of hormonal changes on respiratory function, from an increase in tidal volume to changes in lung capacity. Understand how the body adapts to ensure an efficient exchange of oxygen and carbon dioxide, supporting both the mother and the growing fetus.

2.1.3 Musculoskeletal and Postural Changes

The musculoskeletal system undergoes remarkable changes to accommodate the growing uterus and prepare the body for childbirth. Explore the effects of relaxin and other hormones on ligaments and joints, understanding the importance of these adaptations for the birthing process.

Dive into the alterations in posture and center of gravity, recognizing how these changes may contribute to common discomforts such as back pain. Gain insights into strategies for maintaining musculoskeletal health during pregnancy, from exercises that promote strength and flexibility to ergonomic considerations for daily activities.

2.1.4 Gastrointestinal and Renal Adjustments

Pregnancy brings about notable changes in the gastrointestinal and renal systems, influencing digestion, nutrient absorption, and fluid balance. Explore the effects of hormones such as progesterone on gastrointestinal motility, leading to common symptoms like constipation and heartburn.

Understand the increased workload on the kidneys and the importance of adequate hydration during pregnancy. Delve into the changes in renal function, including alterations in glomerular filtration rate, as the body adapts to support the needs of both the mother and the developing baby.

2.1.5 Endocrine System and Hormonal Symphony

The endocrine system orchestrates a hormonal symphony throughout pregnancy, regulating key processes and ensuring the optimal environment for fetal development. Explore the roles of hormones such as estrogen, progesterone, and oxytocin in maintaining pregnancy and preparing the body for childbirth.

Dive into the endocrine changes that influence metabolic rate, insulin sensitivity, and thyroid function. Understand how these hormonal fluctuations contribute to the energy demands of pregnancy and the regulation of crucial metabolic processes.

2.2 Emotional and Mental Well-being

Pregnancy is not only a physical journey but a profound emotional and mental experience. Understanding and prioritizing emotional well-being is essential for expectant mothers, contributing to a positive pregnancy experience and setting the stage for a healthy transition into motherhood.

2.2.1 Navigating Pregnancy Emotions

The rollercoaster of emotions during pregnancy is a common and natural aspect of the journey. Explore the emotional landscape of pregnancy, from the elation of the first kicks to the occasional bouts of anxiety and mood swings. Understand the role of hormonal fluctuations in influencing emotions and learn strategies for managing and embracing this emotional spectrum.

Delve into the concept of prenatal bonding, exploring ways for expectant parents to connect with the growing baby and each other. From talking to the baby to creating a supportive emotional environment, gain insights into fostering a positive emotional connection throughout pregnancy.

2.2.2 Addressing Mental Health Challenges

Pregnancy may also bring forth mental health challenges, from heightened stress levels to conditions such as prenatal depression and anxiety. Explore the importance of mental health awareness during pregnancy, recognizing the signs of distress and seeking support when needed.

Understand the role of social support, professional counseling, and self-care practices in promoting mental well-being. Delve into mindfulness and relaxation techniques, recognizing their potential to alleviate stress and contribute to a positive emotional state during pregnancy.

2.2.3 Partner Involvement and Communication

The role of partners in supporting the emotional well-being of an expectant mother is paramount. Explore the dynamics of partner involvement during pregnancy, from open communication to active participation in prenatal activities. Understand how partners can provide emotional support, validate feelings, and share in the excitement and challenges of the pregnancy journey.

Delve into the concept of shared responsibility and teamwork, fostering a strong emotional connection between partners. From attending prenatal classes together to creating a supportive birthing plan, gain insights into the various ways partners can actively contribute to the emotional well-being of both the mother and the growing family.

2.2.4 Preparing for the Postpartum Transition

Anticipating the postpartum period is a crucial aspect of emotional well-being during pregnancy. Explore the emotional adjustments that come with the transition to motherhood, from the joy of meeting the baby to the potential challenges of postpartum blues. Understand the importance of realistic expectations and self-compassion during this transformative phase.

Delve into postpartum support systems, recognizing the role of partners, family, and friends in providing emotional assistance. Explore resources for postpartum mental health, understanding when to seek professional help and fostering an open dialogue about the emotional aspects of the postpartum experience.

2.3 Building a Positive Body Image

The changes that accompany pregnancy may present challenges to body image, but fostering a positive and accepting attitude towards one's changing body is crucial for mental and emotional well-being. This section explores strategies for building and maintaining a positive body image throughout the various stages of pregnancy.

2.3.1 Embracing the Changes

Pregnancy brings about physical changes that may challenge traditional notions of beauty and body image. Explore the concept of embracing these changes as a testament to the incredible journey of motherhood. Understand the importance of self-love and self-acceptance, recognizing that a changing body is a powerful vessel supporting the creation of life.

Delve into positive affirmations and mindfulness practices that promote body acceptance, fostering a deep connection with the growing baby and a sense of appreciation for the body's resilience. Learn from the experiences of other mothers who have embraced and celebrated their changing bodies.

2.3.2 Clothing and Self-Expression

The way clothing fits and feels during pregnancy plays a significant role in shaping body image. Explore strategies for dressing comfortably and stylishly during pregnancy, understanding how clothing choices can positively impact self-esteem. Delve into the world of maternity fashion, recognizing the importance of self-expression and feeling good in one's own skin.

Learn about the versatility of maternity clothing, from adaptive fashion choices to embracing body-positive styles that celebrate the pregnant form. Explore the concept of a maternity wardrobe that aligns with personal preferences, fostering a positive and confident self-image.

2.3.3 Pregnancy and Beauty Standards

Pregnancy challenges conventional beauty standards, inviting expectant mothers to redefine their notions of beauty. Delve into the societal expectations surrounding pregnancy and body image, understanding the importance of breaking free from unrealistic standards. Explore the concept of self-defined beauty, where the uniqueness of the pregnant body is celebrated and valued.

Challenge stereotypes and myths surrounding pregnancy and appearance, recognizing that beauty is diverse and multifaceted. Gain insights into reframing beauty standards to align with the authentic and transformative experience of pregnancy.

2.3.4 Partner Support and Communication

Partner support plays a pivotal role in building and maintaining a positive body image during pregnancy. Explore the ways in which partners can actively contribute to promoting body positivity and self-esteem. Understand the importance of open communication, validation, and reassurance in fostering a healthy body image.

Delve into the concept of shared experiences, where partners can express admiration for the changes in the pregnant body and actively participate in promoting body confidence. Gain insights into communication strategies that strengthen the emotional connection between partners, contributing to a positive and supportive environment.

CHAPTER 3

Safe and Effective Exercise During Pregnancy

3.1 Tailoring Workouts to Your Fitness Level

Embarking on a fitness journey during pregnancy is a powerful way to support your overall well-being. However, the key to a safe and effective exercise routine lies in tailoring workouts to your unique fitness level. In this section, we'll explore the importance of understanding and adapting exercises based on your individual fitness capabilities during pregnancy.

3.1.1 Assessing Your Fitness Level

Before delving into a prenatal exercise routine, it's crucial to assess your current fitness level. Understand the components of fitness, including cardiovascular endurance, muscular strength, flexibility, and balance. Evaluate your pre-pregnancy fitness routine and any modifications required due to the changing demands on your body.

Explore the concept of the Borg Rating of Perceived Exertion (RPE) scale, a subjective measure of exercise intensity that allows you to gauge your effort level. Learn how to listen to your body and recognize signs of fatigue or discomfort, ensuring a safe and gradual progression in your fitness journey.

3.1.2 Designing a Customized Exercise Plan

Tailoring workouts to your fitness level involves designing a customized exercise plan that aligns with your goals and physical condition. Explore the components of a well-rounded prenatal exercise routine, encompassing cardiovascular exercises, strength training, flexibility exercises, and balance activities.

Understand the importance of a gradual progression, especially if you were not previously engaged in regular exercise. Learn how to modify intensity, duration, and frequency based on your comfort level and any specific guidelines provided by your healthcare provider. By crafting a personalized plan, you ensure that your exercise routine is both enjoyable and suitable for your individual needs.

3.1.3 Adapting to Physical Changes

Pregnancy brings about unique physical changes that may require adjustments to your exercise routine. Delve into modifications for exercises that involve lying on your back or stomach, considering the changing anatomy of the abdomen. Explore alternative positions and variations that accommodate the growing belly and minimize stress on the lower back.

Understand the impact of the hormone relaxing on joint flexibility and how it influences exercise choices. Learn how to adapt strength training exercises to maintain muscle tone without compromising joint stability. By staying attuned to your body's signals and making necessary adaptations, you can continue to enjoy the benefits of exercise while safeguarding your well-being during pregnancy.

3.1.4 Monitoring Intensity and Heart Rate

One key aspect of tailoring workouts to your fitness level is monitoring exercise intensity and heart rate. Understand the target heart rate zone for pregnant women and how it correlates with the perceived exertion level. Explore the concept of the talk test, a practical way to ensure that you're exercising at a moderate intensity without overexertion.

Learn about heart rate monitors and their applicability during pregnancy, providing real-time feedback on your cardiovascular effort. Delve into the importance of staying within safe intensity ranges, avoiding extremes that could potentially compromise the well-being of both you and your baby. By incorporating heart rate monitoring into your routine, you enhance the safety and effectiveness of your prenatal workouts.

3.2 Prenatal Yoga and Its Benefits

Prenatal yoga emerges as a gentle yet powerful form of exercise that caters specifically to the unique needs of pregnant women. In this section, we'll explore the world of prenatal yoga, its myriad benefits, and how it contributes to a safe and fulfilling exercise regimen during pregnancy.

3.2.1 The Foundations of Prenatal Yoga

Prenatal yoga is rooted in the principles of traditional yoga but is thoughtfully adapted to accommodate the physical changes and needs of expectant mothers. Explore the foundational aspects of prenatal yoga, including gentle stretching, controlled breathing (pranayama), and relaxation techniques. Understand how these elements collectively contribute to improved flexibility, reduced stress, and enhanced well-being during pregnancy.

Learn about the significance of pelvic floor exercises in prenatal yoga, promoting pelvic floor strength and stability. Delve into the modifications made to classic yoga poses to ensure comfort and safety, fostering a practice that nurtures both body and mind.

3.2.2 Physical and Emotional Benefits of Prenatal Yoga

The practice of prenatal yoga extends beyond physical exercise, offering a range of benefits for both the body and the mind. Explore the physical advantages, including improved flexibility, strength, and balance. Understand how prenatal yoga can alleviate common discomforts such as back pain, swelling, and insomnia, fostering a more comfortable pregnancy experience.

Dive into the emotional and mental benefits of prenatal yoga, from stress reduction to enhanced mindfulness. Learn how controlled breathing techniques can be applied during labor, contributing to a more relaxed and focused birthing experience. Through the holistic approach of prenatal yoga, expectant mothers can cultivate a positive mindset and emotional resilience.

3.2.3 Safe and Appropriate Prenatal Yoga Poses

Navigating the world of prenatal yoga involves understanding which poses are safe and appropriate during pregnancy. Explore a variety of yoga poses tailored to the needs of expectant mothers, focusing on those that enhance flexibility, strengthen key muscle groups, and promote relaxation.

Delve into modified versions of common yoga poses, such as downward dog, warrior poses, and twists, ensuring that they are accessible and comfortable for pregnant women. Understand the importance of avoiding deep backbends, inversions, and poses that involve lying flat on the back, considering the potential impact on blood flow and abdominal pressure.

3.2.4 Incorporating Prenatal Yoga Into Your Routine

Incorporating prenatal yoga into your exercise routine involves creating a consistent and enjoyable practice. Explore practical tips for integrating prenatal yoga into your daily life, whether through attending classes, following online sessions, or designing a home practice. Understand the role of props, such as bolsters and blocks, in enhancing comfort and providing additional support during yoga sessions.

Learn about the importance of warm-up and cool-down sequences in prenatal yoga, preparing the body for practice and promoting relaxation afterward. Delve into the concept of mindfulness and present-moment awareness during yoga sessions, fostering a deeper connection with your body and the growing baby.

3.3 Incorporating Cardiovascular Exercise Safely

Cardiovascular exercise is a cornerstone of a well-rounded fitness routine, even during pregnancy. In this section, we'll explore the importance of incorporating cardiovascular exercise safely into your prenatal workouts, reaping the benefits of improved circulation, heart health, and overall vitality.

3.3.1 The Importance of Cardiovascular Exercise in Pregnancy

Cardiovascular exercise offers a range of benefits for both the expectant mother and the growing baby. Explore the importance of maintaining cardiovascular health during pregnancy, including improved circulation, heart function, and stamina. Understand how regular cardiovascular exercise contributes to weight management, reduced pregnancy-related discomforts, and enhanced mood.

Dive into the role of cardiovascular exercise in preparing the body for the physical demands of labor and childbirth. Learn about the potential impact on fetal development and how a healthy maternal cardiovascular system positively influences the baby's well-being.

3.3.2 Safe Forms of Cardiovascular Exercise

Not all forms of cardiovascular exercise are created equal, especially during pregnancy. Delve into safe and effective forms of cardiovascular exercise suitable for expectant mothers. Explore low-impact options, such as walking and swimming, that minimize stress on the joints while providing an effective cardiovascular workout.

Understand the benefits of stationary cycling and elliptical training, offering a combination of cardiovascular exercise and lower-body strengthening. Explore the concept of interval training, where short bursts of higher intensity are alternated with periods of lower intensity, providing cardiovascular benefits without excessive strain.

3.3.3 Monitoring Intensity and Duration

Safe cardiovascular exercise during pregnancy involves a mindful approach to monitoring intensity and duration. Delve into the concept of the talk test as a practical guide to ensure that you're exercising at a moderate intensity without overexertion. Explore the role of perceived exertion and heart rate monitoring in tailoring the intensity of your cardiovascular workouts.

Understand the importance of warm-up and cool-down periods in cardiovascular exercise, preparing the body for activity and promoting a gradual return to rest. Learn how to adjust the duration of your workouts based on your fitness level, allowing for a safe and enjoyable cardiovascular exercise routine throughout pregnancy.

3.3.4 Addressing Safety Precautions and Considerations

While cardiovascular exercise is generally safe during pregnancy, certain precautions and considerations should be kept in mind. Explore safety guidelines, including the importance of staying hydrated, avoiding overheating, and wearing appropriate clothing. Understand the impact of hormonal changes on ligaments and joints, necessitating extra care during activities that involve changes in direction or impact.

Delve into the concept of balance and stability during cardiovascular exercise, especially as the body undergoes changes in center of gravity. Learn about modifications for activities such as aerobics and dance to ensure safety and minimize the risk of falls or injury. By adhering to safety precautions and staying attuned to your body's signals, you can confidently incorporate cardiovascular exercise into your prenatal fitness routine.

CHAPTER 4

Fitness Through Each Trimester

4.1 First Trimester: Building a Foundation

The first trimester of pregnancy is a crucial period marked by the initial stages of fetal development and adjustments in the mother's body. Establishing a solid foundation for fitness during this trimester sets the tone for a healthy and active pregnancy journey. In this section, we'll explore the considerations, exercises, and practices that contribute to building a strong fitness foundation in the first trimester.

4.1.1 Navigating Early Pregnancy Symptoms

The first trimester often brings with it a range of symptoms, including nausea, fatigue, and heightened sensitivity to smells. Explore strategies for adapting your fitness routine to accommodate these symptoms, ensuring a gentle and supportive approach to exercise during this time.

Understand the importance of listening to your body, acknowledging any signs of fatigue, and making necessary modifications to your exercise intensity and duration. Embrace the concept of intuitive fitness, where your routine aligns with your energy levels and well-being.

4.1.2 Gentle Cardiovascular Exercise

Cardiovascular exercise in the first trimester lays the foundation for enhanced circulation, increased energy levels, and overall well-being. Explore low-impact options such as brisk walking, swimming, or stationary cycling, adapting the intensity to suit your comfort level.

Delve into the benefits of cardiovascular exercise for combating fatigue and supporting emotional well-being. Understand the role of warming up and cooling down, ensuring a gradual transition into and out of your cardio workouts. By incorporating gentle cardiovascular exercise, you promote a healthy cardiovascular system and set the stage for continued activity throughout pregnancy.

4.1.3 Core Strengthening and Pelvic Floor Exercises

Building core strength and engaging in pelvic floor exercises form essential components of fitness in the first trimester. Explore safe and effective exercises that target the core without placing undue stress on the abdominal muscles. Learn about modified planks, pelvic tilts, and exercises using stability balls to enhance core stability.

Understand the significance of pelvic floor exercises in promoting pelvic health and preparing for labor. Explore Kegel exercises and other techniques that strengthen the pelvic floor muscles, contributing to bladder control and reducing the risk of pelvic floor issues.

4.1.4 Flexibility and Stretching

Maintaining flexibility is crucial during pregnancy, especially in the first trimester when hormonal changes can impact joint function. Explore gentle stretching exercises that target major muscle groups, promoting flexibility and reducing the risk of muscle tightness.

Learn about the importance of dynamic stretching as part of your warm-up routine, preparing the muscles for activity. Delve into static stretching, incorporating relaxation techniques to enhance flexibility and alleviate tension. By prioritizing flexibility in the first trimester, you support joint health and ensure a well-rounded fitness routine.

4.1.5 Mind-Body Connection and Relaxation Practices

The mind-body connection becomes increasingly important during the first trimester as you adapt to the changes in your body. Explore relaxation practices such as prenatal yoga and mindfulness meditation, fostering a sense of calm and reducing stress.

Understand how deep breathing exercises contribute to relaxation and stress relief. Explore guided imagery and visualization techniques that promote a positive mindset and emotional well-being. By incorporating mind-body practices, you not only enhance your fitness routine but also nurture a holistic approach to well-being during the early stages of pregnancy.

4.2 Second Trimester: Strengthening and Balance

The second trimester is often referred to as the "golden period" of pregnancy, marked by reduced symptoms and increased energy levels. It is an opportune time to focus on strengthening exercises and balance activities that support the changing needs of the body. In this section, we'll delve into effective strategies and exercises for building strength and enhancing balance during the second trimester.

4.2.1 Adjusting Exercise Intensity and Volume

With the alleviation of some first-trimester symptoms, the second trimester allows for a more dynamic and varied fitness routine. Explore strategies for adjusting exercise intensity and volume, incorporating a mix of cardiovascular exercise, strength training, and flexibility activities.

Understand the importance of monitoring your body's response to exercise and making gradual adjustments based on your comfort level. Learn about the benefits of maintaining a well-rounded fitness routine that addresses different aspects of physical health.

4.2.2 Strength Training for the Changing Body

The second trimester presents an opportunity to focus on strength training exercises that accommodate the changing demands on your body. Explore safe and effective strength training exercises that target major muscle groups while considering modifications for comfort and safety.

Understand the role of resistance training using body weight, resistance bands, or light weights to build and maintain muscle tone. Delve into exercises that strengthen the back, legs, and arms, supporting overall posture and reducing the risk of common discomforts such as back pain.

4.2.3 Balance and Stability Workouts

As your body undergoes physical changes, maintaining balance and stability becomes paramount. Explore exercises that enhance balance and stability, incorporating elements of proprioception and coordination. Learn about balance exercises using stability balls, Bosu balls, and simple proprioceptive drills.

Understand the benefits of balance workouts in preventing falls and promoting overall stability. Explore modified yoga poses that focus on balance, adapting them to suit your changing center of gravity. By incorporating balance exercises, you enhance proprioception and reduce the risk of accidents or injuries.

4.2.4 Pelvic Floor Strengthening Continuation

Building on the foundation laid in the first trimester, the second trimester is an ideal time to continue pelvic floor strengthening exercises. Explore progressive Kegel exercises and variations that challenge the pelvic floor muscles in different ways.

Understand the role of pelvic floor exercises in preventing and addressing common issues such as urinary incontinence. Learn how to integrate pelvic floor exercises into your daily routine, ensuring consistency and effectiveness. By prioritizing pelvic floor health, you contribute to overall core strength and stability.

4.2.5 Cardiovascular Challenges and Solutions

Cardiovascular exercise continues to be an essential component of fitness in the second trimester, but adjustments may be needed as your body changes. Explore strategies for addressing cardiovascular challenges, such as changes in balance and potential discomfort.

Understand the benefits of low-impact cardio exercises, including swimming and stationary cycling, to reduce stress on the joints. Delve into modifications for high-impact activities, ensuring a safe and enjoyable cardiovascular workout. By adapting your cardio routine, you maintain cardiovascular health while prioritizing safety and comfort.

4.3 Third Trimester: Gentle Movement and Preparation for Birth

The third trimester heralds the final stages of pregnancy, and as the body prepares for childbirth, the focus shifts to gentle movement, preparation for labor, and relaxation. In this section, we'll explore safe and effective strategies for maintaining fitness during the third trimester, considering the unique challenges and opportunities this stage presents.

4.3.1 Embracing Gentle Movement and Low-Impact Cardio

As the body undergoes significant changes in the third trimester, embracing gentle movement becomes key to maintaining fitness. Explore low-impact cardiovascular exercises that prioritize comfort and safety, such as walking, swimming, and prenatal dance.

Understand the benefits of water-based activities, which provide buoyancy and reduce the impact on joints. Delve into the concept of listening to your body and adjusting the intensity of your workouts to align with your energy levels. By incorporating gentle movement, you promote circulation, alleviate discomfort, and support overall well-being.

4.3.2 Prenatal Yoga and Relaxation Practices

Prenatal yoga takes center stage in the third trimester, offering a combination of gentle movement, stretching, and relaxation. Explore modified yoga poses that cater to the changing needs of the body, with a focus on comfort and ease. Learn about poses that encourage optimal fetal positioning and preparation for labor.

Delve into relaxation practices within prenatal yoga, including guided meditation and deep breathing exercises. Understand the role of mindfulness in reducing stress and promoting a positive mindset as you approach childbirth. By embracing prenatal yoga and relaxation techniques, you create a supportive and nurturing environment for both you and your baby.

4.3.3 Pelvic Floor Exercises and Birthing Positions

The third trimester is a crucial time to continue pelvic floor exercises, with a specific focus on preparing for labor. Explore exercises that strengthen and release the pelvic floor muscles, promoting flexibility and resilience. Learn about the benefits of perineal massage and its potential impact on reducing the risk of tearing during childbirth.

Delve into birthing positions and movements that align with your body's natural processes. Understand the advantages of upright positions, squatting, and using birthing balls during labor. Explore how pelvic floor exercises contribute to the ability to engage and relax the pelvic floor muscles, facilitating a smoother birthing experience.

4.3.4 Strength Maintenance and Adaptations
While the focus in the third trimester shifts towards gentle movement, it's important to maintain overall strength to support daily activities. Explore modified strength training exercises that prioritize comfort and safety. Learn about exercises that engage major muscle groups while avoiding positions that may strain the abdominal muscles.

Understand the benefits of bodyweight exercises and resistance band workouts in maintaining muscle tone. Delve into adaptations for common strength training exercises, ensuring they align with the changing needs of your body. By continuing to engage in strength maintenance, you support functional fitness and ease of movement in daily life.

4.3.5 Preparation for Postpartum Recovery

The third trimester is a transitional phase that sets the stage for postpartum recovery. Explore exercises and practices that contribute to a smoother recovery period. Learn about perineal stretches and pelvic floor exercises that support tissue elasticity and healing.

Delve into the importance of maintaining mobility and flexibility, incorporating gentle stretches and movements. Understand the role of deep breathing exercises in promoting relaxation and reducing tension. By actively preparing for postpartum recovery, you contribute to the overall well-being of both you and your baby.

CHAPTER 5

Postpartum Fitness Journey

5.1 Easing Back into Exercise After Birth

The postpartum period marks a transformative phase in a woman's life, and as the body undergoes recovery, re-engaging with exercise requires a thoughtful and gradual approach. In this section, we'll explore the importance of easing back into exercise after birth, addressing physical and emotional considerations to support a healthy and sustainable postpartum fitness journey.

5.1.1 Understanding Postpartum Recovery

The first weeks and months after giving birth are dedicated to postpartum recovery, a period in which the body heals and adjusts to the changes brought about by pregnancy and childbirth. Explore the physical aspects of recovery, including uterine involution, healing of perineal tissues, and hormonal adjustments.

Understand the emotional and mental components of postpartum recovery, recognizing the significance of rest, self-care, and bonding with the newborn. Delve into the concept of embracing the body's natural timeline for recovery, understanding that every woman's journey is unique.

5.1.2 Listening to Your Body

Easing back into exercise after birth begins with a keen awareness of your body's signals and needs. Explore the importance of listening to your body during the postpartum period, recognizing signs of fatigue, discomfort, or overexertion.

Understand the role of hormonal changes, breastfeeding, and sleep patterns in influencing your energy levels and recovery. Delve into the concept of intuitive exercise, where you adjust the intensity and duration of workouts based on how you feel on a given day. By cultivating a mindful and responsive approach, you lay the foundation for a positive postpartum fitness experience.

5.1.3 Incorporating Gentle Movement

Gentle movement forms the cornerstone of easing back into exercise after birth. Explore postpartum-friendly activities such as walking, pelvic floor exercises, and gentle stretching. Learn about the benefits of low-impact exercises in promoting circulation, reducing muscle tension, and supporting overall well-being.

Delve into postpartum yoga, a practice that combines gentle movement with mindfulness and relaxation. Understand how modified yoga poses can contribute to pelvic floor recovery, improved flexibility, and a gradual return to physical activity. By incorporating gentle movement, you provide your body with the opportunity to rebuild strength while respecting its postpartum needs.

5.1.4 Core and Pelvic Floor Restoration

The postpartum period often brings changes to the core and pelvic floor muscles, necessitating a focused approach to restoration. Explore exercises that target core strength without placing undue stress on the abdominal muscles. Learn about pelvic floor exercises that promote recovery and enhance pelvic health.

Understand the importance of re-establishing a connection with the core and pelvic floor muscles, incorporating breathwork and gentle contractions. Delve into exercises that address diastasis recti, a common postpartum condition where the abdominal muscles separate. By prioritizing core and pelvic floor restoration, you lay the groundwork for a strong and functional foundation.

5.1.5 Gradual Progression and Patience

Easing back into exercise after birth requires a gradual and patient approach. Explore strategies for progressive exercise, starting with low-intensity activities and gradually increasing the intensity and duration as your body adapts. Learn about the importance of pacing yourself and avoiding the temptation to rush into more intense workouts.

Understand that postpartum recovery is a dynamic process, and your fitness routine should evolve alongside your changing needs. Delve into the concept of setting realistic expectations and celebrating small milestones in your postpartum fitness journey. By embracing gradual progression and practicing patience, you support a sustainable and positive return to regular exercise.

5.2 Targeted Workouts for Postpartum Recovery

As the postpartum journey unfolds, targeted workouts play a vital role in restoring strength, flexibility, and overall fitness. In this section, we'll explore specific exercises and workouts designed to support postpartum recovery, addressing key areas such as the core, pelvic floor, and overall muscular strength.

5.2.1 Core-Strengthening Exercises

Restoring core strength is a focal point of postpartum recovery, and targeted exercises can aid in this process. Explore postpartum-friendly core exercises that engage the abdominal muscles without straining the midsection.

Learn about modified versions of traditional core exercises, such as pelvic tilts, seated leg lifts, and gentle planks. Understand the importance of focusing on the deeper core muscles, including the transverse abdominis, to promote stability and support the lower back. By incorporating targeted core exercises, you contribute to the gradual restoration of abdominal strength.

5.2.2 Pelvic Floor Strengthening Workouts

Pelvic floor strength is integral to postpartum recovery, especially after the strain of childbirth. Explore targeted workouts that focus on pelvic floor engagement and strengthening.

Learn about Kegel exercises and variations that address different aspects of pelvic floor function. Understand how breathwork can be integrated into pelvic floor exercises to enhance coordination and relaxation. Delve into the concept of progressive resistance, gradually increasing the intensity of pelvic floor workouts over time. By prioritizing pelvic floor strengthening, you support urinary and pelvic health in the postpartum period.

5.2.3 Full-Body Strength Training

Comprehensive postpartum recovery involves full-body strength training to rebuild overall muscular strength and endurance. Explore exercises that target major muscle groups, including the legs, arms, and back.

Learn about resistance training using body weight, resistance bands, or light weights to provide a controlled and gradual challenge. Understand the importance of maintaining proper form and alignment to prevent injury and support joint health. Delve into modified versions of classic strength training exercises, ensuring they align with your postpartum fitness goals. By incorporating full-body strength training, you foster a balanced and functional recovery.

5.2.4 Flexibility and Mobility Routines

Flexibility and mobility play key roles in postpartum recovery, promoting joint health and reducing muscle tension. Explore targeted routines that focus on stretching major muscle groups, improving flexibility, and addressing common postpartum discomforts.

Learn about dynamic stretching as part of your warm-up routine and static stretching for relaxation and enhanced range of motion. Understand the benefits of incorporating yoga or Pilates into your postpartum fitness routine, combining flexibility exercises with mindful movement. By prioritizing flexibility and mobility, you enhance overall physical well-being and support your body's recovery.

5.2.5 Cardiovascular Exercise in the Postpartum Period

Cardiovascular exercise is a valuable component of postpartum recovery, contributing to improved circulation, energy levels, and overall cardiovascular health. Explore postpartum-friendly cardiovascular activities that prioritize comfort and safety.

Learn about low-impact options such as brisk walking, swimming, or stationary cycling, adapting the intensity to suit your postpartum fitness level. Understand the benefits of interval training, allowing for variations in intensity and duration. Delve into the concept of gradual progression, starting with shorter sessions and gradually increasing both time and intensity. By incorporating cardiovascular exercise, you support overall health and contribute to a well-rounded postpartum fitness routine.

5.3 Establishing a Sustainable Fitness Routine

As postpartum recovery progresses, establishing a sustainable fitness routine becomes paramount for long-term well-being. In this section, we'll explore strategies for creating a balanced and realistic postpartum fitness routine that aligns with your lifestyle and evolving needs.

5.3.1 Assessing Time and Energy Constraints

The postpartum period brings unique time and energy constraints, requiring a realistic assessment of your daily schedule and available resources. Explore strategies for adapting your fitness routine to accommodate the demands of caring for a newborn, potential sleep disruptions, and other responsibilities.

Understand the concept of "micro workouts," incorporating short and focused exercise sessions throughout the day. Learn about the benefits of prioritizing consistency over duration, allowing for flexibility in your fitness routine. By assessing time and energy constraints, you create a sustainable framework for postpartum fitness.

5.3.2 Integrating Exercise into Daily Activities

Incorporating exercise into daily activities is a practical approach to postpartum fitness. Explore strategies for seamlessly integrating movement into tasks such as baby care, household chores, and outdoor activities.

Learn about exercises that can be performed while carrying or interacting with your baby, fostering a sense of connection and bonding. Understand the benefits of postpartum-friendly activities such as stroller walks, babywearing workouts, and gentle yoga stretches. By making exercise an integral part of your daily routine, you cultivate a sustainable and enjoyable approach to postpartum fitness.

5.3.3 Setting Realistic and Achievable Goals

Setting realistic and achievable goals is essential for postpartum fitness success. Explore the concept of SMART goals—specific, measurable, achievable, relevant, and time-bound—as a framework for goal setting.

Understand the importance of focusing on progress rather than perfection, celebrating small victories along the way. Learn about the dynamic nature of postpartum fitness goals, adjusting them as your body and lifestyle evolve. Delve into the concept of self-compassion, acknowledging the challenges of the postpartum period and embracing a positive mindset toward your fitness journey.

5.3.4 Seeking Support and Accountability

Building a postpartum fitness routine is often enhanced by seeking support and accountability. Explore strategies for involving a workout buddy, whether it's a friend, partner, or fellow postpartum mom.

Learn about the benefits of joining postpartum fitness classes or online communities, creating a supportive network that shares experiences and tips. Understand the role of professional guidance, such as postpartum fitness trainers or physical therapists, in tailoring a routine to your specific needs. By seeking support and accountability, you enhance motivation and foster a sense of community in your postpartum fitness journey.

5.3.5 Adapting to Changing Needs

The postpartum period is characterized by evolving needs, and adapting your fitness routine accordingly is crucial for long-term success. Explore strategies for modifying your workouts based on factors such as changes in sleep patterns, postpartum recovery milestones, and shifting priorities.

Understand the concept of periodization, which involves organizing your fitness routine into distinct phases to address different goals and challenges. Learn about the flexibility of exercise modalities, allowing you to explore new activities or modify existing ones as needed. By embracing adaptability, you create a sustainable postpartum fitness routine that aligns with the dynamic nature of this transformative period.

CHAPTER 6

Nourishing Your Body and Baby

6.1 Importance of a Balanced Diet During Pregnancy

The journey of pregnancy is a remarkable and transformative period, and proper nutrition plays a pivotal role in supporting both the mother's well-being and the optimal development of the growing baby. In this section, we'll delve into the importance of maintaining a balanced diet during pregnancy, exploring the key nutrients and dietary considerations essential for a healthy and thriving pregnancy.

6.1.1 Foundation of a Healthy Pregnancy Diet

A balanced diet during pregnancy serves as the foundation for ensuring the health and well-being of both the expectant mother and the developing baby. Explore the concept of balance in the context of pregnancy nutrition, emphasizing the importance of incorporating a variety of food groups to meet the diverse nutritional needs.

Understand the role of macronutrients—carbohydrates, proteins, and fats—in providing essential energy and building blocks for fetal development. Delve into the significance of micronutrients—vitamins and minerals—in supporting various physiological processes and preventing nutritional deficiencies. By embracing a well-rounded and diverse diet, you create an environment that fosters optimal growth and development during pregnancy.

6.1.2 Caloric Intake and Energy Needs

The caloric intake during pregnancy is a critical consideration, ensuring that the expectant mother consumes an appropriate amount of energy to support both her own needs and the demands of fetal growth. Explore the concept of increased energy needs during pregnancy, influenced by factors such as maternal weight, physical activity level, and stage of pregnancy.

Understand how caloric requirements evolve throughout each trimester, recognizing the dynamic nature of energy needs. Delve into the concept of mindful eating, where the emphasis is on the quality of calories consumed, ensuring they contribute to both nutritional needs and overall well-being. By understanding and meeting appropriate caloric intake, you contribute to a healthy and balanced pregnancy.

6.1.3 Importance of Hydration

Hydration is a fundamental aspect of a balanced pregnancy diet, supporting various bodily functions and contributing to overall health. Explore the importance of adequate water intake during pregnancy, recognizing that hydration needs may increase due to physiological changes and increased blood volume.

Understand the benefits of water in promoting digestion, nutrient transport, and temperature regulation. Delve into strategies for staying hydrated, including regular water consumption, herbal teas, and the incorporation of water-rich foods. By prioritizing hydration, you support optimal physiological function and create a foundation for a healthy pregnancy.

6.1.4 Role of Fiber in Pregnancy Nutrition

Dietary fiber plays a crucial role in pregnancy nutrition, promoting digestive health, managing weight, and preventing constipation—an often-common concern during pregnancy. Explore the sources of dietary fiber, including fruits, vegetables, whole grains, and legumes, and understand their significance in maintaining gastrointestinal health.

Learn about the recommended daily intake of fiber during pregnancy and practical ways to incorporate fiber-rich foods into meals and snacks. Delve into the benefits of fiber in managing blood sugar levels, supporting satiety, and contributing to overall nutritional balance. By emphasizing fiber in the pregnancy diet, you enhance digestive well-being and ensure the efficient absorption of nutrients.

6.2 Key Nutrients for Mom and Baby

Ensuring adequate intake of key nutrients is a cornerstone of a healthy pregnancy, influencing the development of the baby's organs, tissues, and overall well-being. In this section, we'll explore the essential nutrients for both the expectant mother and the growing baby, understanding their roles and sources in promoting a thriving pregnancy.

6.2.1 Folate and Folic Acid

Folate, a B-vitamin, is a vital nutrient during pregnancy, playing a crucial role in the early development of the baby's neural tube. Explore the importance of folate in preventing neural tube defects, such as spina bifida, and understand the difference between dietary folate and folic acid, a synthetic form often found in supplements and fortified foods.

Learn about folate-rich foods, including leafy green vegetables, legumes, and fortified grains, and understand the recommended daily intake during pregnancy. Delve into the significance of folate supplementation, especially in the early stages of pregnancy, to ensure optimal neural tube development and overall fetal health.

6.2.2 Iron for Hemoglobin Production

Iron is a key nutrient that becomes especially important during pregnancy due to increased blood volume and the development of the baby's blood supply. Explore the role of iron in hemoglobin production, which is essential for transporting oxygen to both the mother and the developing baby.

Understand the sources of dietary iron, including lean meats, poultry, fish, beans, and fortified cereals. Delve into factors that influence iron absorption, such as vitamin C-rich foods, and recognize the importance of iron supplementation when needed. By prioritizing iron intake, you support the prevention of iron-deficiency anemia and contribute to optimal oxygen transport during pregnancy.

6.2.3 Calcium for Bone Development

Calcium is a vital nutrient for supporting the development of the baby's bones, teeth, and overall skeletal structure during pregnancy. Explore the importance of calcium in preventing maternal bone loss and supporting the growing baby's mineralization process.

Understand dietary sources of calcium, including dairy products, leafy green vegetables, and fortified plant-based milk alternatives. Delve into strategies for meeting calcium needs, especially for individuals with dietary restrictions or preferences. Recognize the role of vitamin D in calcium absorption and the potential need for supplementation. By ensuring adequate calcium intake, you contribute to the formation of a strong skeletal foundation for the baby.

6.2.4 Omega-3 Fatty Acids for Brain Development

Omega-3 fatty acids, particularly docosahexaenoic acid (DHA), are critical for the development of the baby's brain and nervous system. Explore the sources of omega-3 fatty acids, including fatty fish, walnuts, and flaxseeds, and understand their role in promoting cognitive function and visual development.

Learn about the potential benefits of omega-3 supplementation during pregnancy, especially for individuals with limited dietary intake. Delve into considerations for choosing high-quality omega-3 supplements and recognizing the importance of balance with omega-6 fatty acids. By prioritizing omega-3 fatty acids, you support the neurodevelopmental aspects of the growing baby.

6.2.5 Protein for Growth and Tissue Repair

Protein is a fundamental nutrient for supporting the overall growth and development of the baby's tissues, organs, and muscles. Explore the importance of protein in pregnancy, understanding its role in cellular function, immune system support, and tissue repair.

Understand dietary sources of protein, including lean meats, poultry, fish, eggs, dairy products, legumes, and plant-based protein sources. Delve into considerations for meeting increased protein needs during pregnancy, especially in the second and third trimesters. Recognize the importance of variety in protein sources to ensure a diverse amino acid profile. By prioritizing protein intake, you contribute to the building blocks necessary for the baby's growth and development.

6.3 Addressing Common Nutritional Concerns

Pregnancy often brings about specific nutritional concerns and challenges, ranging from managing weight gain to addressing potential deficiencies. In this section, we'll explore common nutritional concerns during pregnancy and strategies for maintaining optimal health for both the expectant mother and the growing baby.

6.3.1 Managing Healthy Weight Gain

Healthy weight gain during pregnancy is a key aspect of ensuring the well-being of both the mother and the baby. Explore the concept of appropriate weight gain based on pre-pregnancy body mass index (BMI) and individual factors. Understand the distribution of weight gain throughout each trimester and the specific considerations for multiple pregnancies.

Learn about the importance of nutrient-dense foods in supporting healthy weight gain and avoiding excessive calorie intake from empty-calorie foods. Delve into strategies for addressing common pregnancy cravings and balancing indulgences with a focus on overall nutrition. By managing healthy weight gain, you support the baby's development and minimize the risk of complications during pregnancy.

6.3.2 Gestational Diabetes and Blood Sugar Management

Gestational diabetes is a condition that can develop during pregnancy, affecting blood sugar levels and requiring careful management through diet and lifestyle. Explore the concept of gestational diabetes, its risk factors, and the importance of regular screening.

Understand dietary strategies for managing blood sugar levels, including balanced meals, portion control, and the distribution of carbohydrates throughout the day. Delve into the significance of regular physical activity in blood sugar management and overall well-being. Recognize the potential need for medication or insulin therapy in cases of gestational diabetes. By addressing blood sugar concerns, you contribute to a healthy pregnancy and minimize the risk of complications for both mother and baby.

6.3.3 Dealing with Nausea and Food Aversions

Nausea and food aversions are common experiences during pregnancy, impacting dietary choices and nutrient intake. Explore strategies for managing nausea and adapting your diet to accommodate food aversions. Understand the importance of small, frequent meals and snacks in alleviating nausea.

Learn about nutritionally dense foods that can be well-tolerated during periods of nausea, including crackers, ginger, and plain yogurt. Delve into the role of hydration and potential modifications to meal preparation to minimize aversions. By navigating nausea and food aversions, you ensure continued access to essential nutrients and support overall well-being during pregnancy.

6.3.4 Addressing Iron Deficiency and Anemia

Iron deficiency and anemia are common concerns during pregnancy, affecting both maternal health and the baby's development. Explore the risk factors for iron deficiency, including increased iron needs during pregnancy and potential dietary sources.

Understand strategies for enhancing iron absorption, such as combining iron-rich foods with vitamin C sources. Delve into considerations for iron supplementation, especially for individuals at higher risk of deficiency. Recognize the importance of monitoring iron levels through regular blood tests and adjusting dietary or supplemental iron intake accordingly. By addressing iron deficiency, you contribute to optimal oxygen transport and overall well-being during pregnancy.

6.3.5 Coping with Dietary Restrictions and Preferences

Dietary restrictions and preferences, whether due to cultural, ethical, or medical reasons, can pose unique challenges during pregnancy. Explore strategies for meeting nutritional needs while adhering to specific dietary choices, such as vegetarianism, veganism, or gluten-free diets.

Understand the importance of careful planning and diverse food choices to ensure a well-rounded nutrient intake. Delve into considerations for potential nutrient deficiencies associated with specific dietary restrictions and the role of supplements in filling potential gaps. Recognize the importance of open communication with healthcare providers to address any concerns or questions related to dietary preferences. By navigating dietary restrictions and preferences, you create a supportive and nutritious environment for a healthy pregnancy.

CHAPTER 7

The First-Time Mom's Cookbook

7.1 Quick and Healthy Meal Planning Tips

Meal planning is a crucial aspect of maintaining a healthy and balanced diet during pregnancy, especially for first-time moms navigating the challenges of pregnancy. In this section, we'll explore practical and efficient meal planning tips tailored to the unique needs of expectant mothers, emphasizing quick and nutritious options that support both maternal well-being and the optimal development of the growing baby.

7.1.1 Importance of Meal Planning During Pregnancy

Meal planning during pregnancy serves as a valuable tool for ensuring consistent access to nourishing and well-balanced meals. Explore the specific considerations that make meal planning essential for first-time moms, including managing energy levels, addressing nutritional needs, and minimizing stress associated with meal preparation.

Understand how meal planning contributes to the prevention of unhealthy food choices and the promotion of a diverse and nutrient-rich diet. Delve into the time-saving benefits of meal planning, providing more opportunities for rest, self-care, and relaxation during pregnancy. By recognizing the importance of meal planning, first-time moms can cultivate a supportive and sustainable approach to nutrition.

7.1.2 Quick and Nutrient-Dense Ingredients

Efficiency is key in meal planning for first-time moms, and selecting quick and nutrient-dense ingredients forms the foundation of time-effective and health-conscious meals. Explore a variety of pantry staples, fresh produce, lean proteins, and whole grains that can be easily incorporated into quick and nutritious recipes.

Learn about the benefits of batch cooking and prepping ingredients in advance, saving time and ensuring a readily available supply of healthy components. Delve into the concept of versatile ingredients that can be used in multiple recipes, promoting variety without excessive complexity. By focusing on quick and nutrient-dense ingredients, first-time moms can streamline their meal preparation while prioritizing nutritional quality.

7.1.3 Balanced Macronutrient Ratios

Maintaining balanced macronutrient ratios is essential for meeting the diverse nutritional needs of pregnancy. Explore the ideal distribution of carbohydrates, proteins, and fats in pregnancy meals, understanding their roles in providing energy, supporting fetal development, and ensuring overall well-being.

Learn about the significance of complex carbohydrates, such as whole grains and legumes, in providing sustained energy and preventing blood sugar fluctuations. Understand the importance of protein sources, including lean meats, dairy, and plant-based options, in promoting tissue repair and fetal growth. Delve into the role of healthy fats, such as those found in avocados, nuts, and olive oil, in supporting brain development and hormone production. By prioritizing balanced macronutrient ratios, first-time moms can optimize their nutritional intake and foster a healthy pregnancy.

7.1.4 Mindful Portion Control

Mindful portion control is a valuable strategy in meal planning, helping first-time moms manage their caloric intake and prevent overeating. Explore practical tips for portion control, including the use of smaller plates, mindful eating practices, and paying attention to hunger and fullness cues.

Learn about the importance of listening to your body's signals during pregnancy, recognizing the dynamic nature of hunger and satiety. Understand the potential impact of hormonal changes on appetite and cravings, emphasizing the role of balanced and satisfying meals. Delve into the concept of nutrient-dense snacks that contribute to overall satiety without excessive caloric intake. By practicing mindful portion control, first-time moms can maintain a healthy weight during pregnancy and support optimal nutrition for both themselves and their babies.

7.1.5 Time-Saving Meal Prep Strategies

Time-saving meal prep strategies are essential for first-time moms juggling the demands of pregnancy, work, and other responsibilities. Explore practical and efficient meal prep techniques, including batch cooking, freezer-friendly recipes, and strategic ingredient prepping.

Learn about the benefits of creating a weekly meal plan, simplifying grocery shopping and minimizing food waste. Understand the role of versatile base ingredients that can be transformed into multiple meals throughout the week. Delve into the concept of designated meal prep days, allowing first-time moms to dedicate specific time slots to preparing ingredients and assembling meals. By incorporating time-saving meal prep strategies, expectant mothers can navigate the challenges of meal planning with ease and efficiency.

7.2 Nutrient-Rich Recipes for Pregnancy

Creating nutrient-rich and delicious meals is a joyful part of the pregnancy journey, and first-time moms can embrace a variety of recipes that cater to their specific nutritional needs. In this section, we'll explore a collection of nutrient-rich recipes designed to provide essential vitamins and minerals, support energy levels, and satisfy taste buds during pregnancy.

7.2.1 Breakfast: Power-Packed Smoothie Bowl

Start the day with a nutrient-packed smoothie bowl that combines a variety of vitamins, minerals, and essential nutrients. Explore the inclusion of vibrant fruits such as berries, banana, and mango for a burst of antioxidants and natural sweetness.

Learn about incorporating leafy greens like spinach or kale for added folate and iron, essential for fetal development. Explore protein sources such as

Greek yogurt or plant-based alternatives, providing a satisfying and energy-boosting breakfast. Delve into creative toppings such as nuts, seeds, and granola for added texture and additional nutritional benefits. By enjoying a power-packed smoothie bowl for breakfast, first-time moms can kickstart their day with a delicious and nutrient-rich meal.

7.2.2 Lunch: Quinoa Salad with Avocado and Chickpeas

For a wholesome and satisfying lunch, consider a quinoa salad loaded with nutrient-rich ingredients. Explore the versatility of quinoa, a complete protein, as the base for the salad, providing essential amino acids for both the mother and the baby.

Learn about incorporating fresh vegetables like cherry tomatoes, cucumber, and bell peppers for a colorful array of vitamins and minerals. Explore the addition of protein-rich chickpeas for sustained energy and satiety. Delve into the creamy goodness of avocado, offering healthy fats and additional folate. By preparing a quinoa salad with avocado and chickpeas, first-time moms can enjoy a delicious and nutritionally balanced lunch.

7.2.3 Dinner: Baked Salmon with Roasted Vegetables

Dinner can be both flavorful and nutritionally dense with a baked salmon dish accompanied by roasted vegetables. Explore the omega-3 fatty acids in salmon, supporting the baby's brain development and offering a high-quality protein source for the mother.

Learn about the variety of vegetables that can be roasted, such as sweet potatoes, broccoli, and carrots, providing a mix of vitamins and minerals. Explore simple seasoning options like lemon, garlic, and herbs for added flavor without excessive sodium. Delve into the convenience of baking, allowing for a hands-off approach to cooking while ensuring a delicious and nutrient-rich dinner. By savoring baked salmon with roasted vegetables, first-time moms can enjoy a dinner that combines taste with essential nutrients.

7.2.4 Snack: Greek Yogurt Parfait with Berries

Snacking becomes an opportunity for nutrient-rich indulgence with a Greek yogurt parfait featuring an assortment of berries. Explore the protein-packed goodness of Greek yogurt, offering calcium for bone health and probiotics for gut health.

Learn about the antioxidant-rich properties of berries such as blueberries, strawberries, and raspberries, contributing to overall well-being. Explore the option of adding a sprinkle of nuts or seeds for an extra crunch and a dose of healthy fats. Delve into the customizable nature of a yogurt parfait, allowing first-time moms to tailor the snack to their taste preferences and nutritional needs. By enjoying a Greek yogurt parfait with berries, expectant mothers can satisfy cravings while supporting their health.

7.2.5 Dessert: Dark Chocolate and Nut Energy Bites

Indulging in a nutrient-dense dessert is a delightful way for first-time moms to satisfy their sweet tooth while incorporating essential nutrients. Explore the creation of dark chocolate and nut energy bites, combining rich flavors with nutritional benefits.

Learn about the health benefits of dark chocolate, including antioxidants and potential mood-boosting properties. Explore the variety of nuts such as almonds, walnuts, and cashews, providing healthy fats, protein, and a range of vitamins and minerals. Delve into the simplicity of creating energy bites, offering a convenient and portion-controlled dessert option. By savoring dark chocolate and nut energy bites, first-time moms can enjoy a guilt-free treat that aligns with their nutritional goals.

7.3 Family-Friendly Meals for Busy Moms

Navigating family-friendly meals while managing the demands of pregnancy and motherhood requires thoughtful planning and consideration. In this section, we'll explore a collection of family-friendly meal ideas that cater to the nutritional needs of expectant mothers, while also appealing to the tastes of the entire family. These meals are designed to be quick, nutritious, and enjoyable for busy moms juggling multiple responsibilities.

7.3.1 One-Pan Chicken and Vegetable Stir-Fry

Simplify dinner preparation with a one-pan chicken and vegetable stir-fry, offering a combination of lean protein and colorful veggies. Explore the versatility of stir-fry by incorporating a mix of broccoli, bell peppers, snap peas, and carrots for a nutrient-packed meal.

Learn about marinating the chicken in a flavorful sauce, infusing the dish with taste without excessive salt or sugar. Explore the option of using brown rice or quinoa as a base for added fiber and sustained energy. Delve into the convenience of one-pan cooking, minimizing cleanup and maximizing efficiency in the kitchen. By preparing a one-pan chicken and vegetable stir-fry, busy moms can deliver a delicious and wholesome meal for the entire family.

7.3.2 Vegetarian Chili with Quinoa

A hearty and nutritious vegetarian chili with quinoa is a family-friendly option that caters to various dietary preferences while offering essential nutrients. Explore the protein-rich goodness of quinoa, complemented by a medley of beans such as black beans, kidney beans, and chickpeas.

Learn about incorporating a variety of vegetables, including tomatoes, onions, and bell peppers, for added vitamins and minerals. Explore the flavorful combination of chili spices, offering taste without excessive sodium. Delve into the option of serving the chili with toppings like shredded cheese, avocado, and Greek yogurt for added texture and flavor. By preparing a vegetarian chili with quinoa, busy moms can create a versatile and nourishing meal for the whole family.

7.3.3 Sheet Pan Salmon with Roasted Potatoes and Asparagus

Sheet pan meals are a time-saving solution for busy moms, and a combination of salmon, roasted potatoes, and asparagus offers a well-rounded and flavorful option. Explore the omega-3 fatty acids in salmon, supporting both maternal and fetal health.

Learn about the convenience of roasting potatoes and asparagus on the same sheet pan, minimizing kitchen cleanup. Explore simple seasoning options such as lemon, garlic, and herbs for added taste. Delve into the versatility of sheet pan cooking, allowing for customization based on family preferences and ingredient availability. By preparing a sheet pan salmon with roasted potatoes and asparagus, busy moms can deliver a nutritious and hassle-free dinner for the entire family.

7.3.4 Whole Wheat Pasta with Spinach and Cherry Tomatoes

A family-friendly pasta dish featuring whole wheat pasta, spinach, and cherry tomatoes provides a quick and wholesome option for busy moms. Explore the nutritional benefits of whole wheat pasta, offering fiber and complex carbohydrates for sustained energy.

Learn about incorporating fresh spinach for added iron, folate, and vitamins. Explore the vibrant burst of flavor from cherry tomatoes, contributing antioxidants and a touch of sweetness. Delve into simple and quick preparation techniques, allowing busy moms to create a satisfying meal without extensive cooking time. By preparing whole wheat pasta with spinach and cherry tomatoes, moms can offer a delicious and nutritious option that appeals to both adults and children.

7.3.5 Grilled Chicken Wrap with Hummus and Vegetables

A grilled chicken wrap with hummus and vegetables is a versatile and handheld option that suits the preferences of family members of all ages. Explore the lean protein in grilled chicken, offering essential amino acids for growth and development.

Learn about the creamy and nutritious addition of hummus, providing a flavorful spread without excessive saturated fats. Explore a varicty of colorful vegetables such as lettuce, cucumbers, and bell peppers for added crunch and vitamins. Delve into the adaptability of wraps, allowing for customization based on individual tastes and dietary restrictions. By preparing grilled chicken wraps with hummus and vegetables, busy moms can offer a customizable and satisfying meal for the entire family.

CHAPTER 8

Balancing Motherhood and Self-Care

8.1 Prioritizing Mental and Emotional Well-being

The journey into motherhood is a transformative experience, marked by joy, challenges, and profound emotional shifts. In this section, we'll delve into the importance of prioritizing mental and emotional well-being for new moms, exploring strategies to navigate the complexities of motherhood while fostering a positive and resilient mindset.

8.1.1 Acknowledging the Emotional Landscape of Motherhood

The emotional landscape of motherhood is diverse and dynamic, encompassing a spectrum of feelings from overwhelming love and joy to moments of self-doubt and stress. Explore the importance of acknowledging and normalizing the range of emotions experienced by new moms, emphasizing that the complexities of motherhood are shared among many.

Understand the impact of hormonal changes, sleep deprivation, and adjusting to a new role on emotional well-being. Delve into the concept of self-compassion, encouraging new moms to be kind to themselves and recognize that it's normal to experience a mix of emotions during this transformative period. By acknowledging the emotional landscape of motherhood, new moms can lay the foundation for prioritizing their mental well-being.

8.1.2 Establishing Open Communication

Open communication, both with oneself and with others, is a cornerstone of prioritizing mental and emotional well-being. Explore strategies for fostering self-reflection, allowing new moms to tune into their feelings, needs, and boundaries.

Learn about the importance of communicating openly with partners, friends, and family members about the challenges and joys of motherhood. Understand the power of expressing emotions and seeking support when needed. Delve into the concept of setting realistic expectations, both for oneself and in terms of societal pressures, fostering a sense of authenticity and openness. By establishing open communication, new moms can create a supportive environment that nurtures their mental and emotional health.

8.1.3 Embracing Self-Compassion Practices

Self-compassion is a powerful practice that can positively impact mental well-being, especially for new moms navigating the demands of motherhood. Explore the components of self-compassion, including self-kindness, common humanity, and mindfulness.

Learn about practical self-compassion exercises, such as positive self-talk, affirmations, and mindfulness meditation, that can be integrated into daily routines. Understand the role of self-care activities in promoting self-compassion, acknowledging that taking time for oneself is not selfish but essential for overall well-being. Delve into the concept of self-forgiveness, recognizing that imperfections are part of the journey and do not diminish one's worth as a mother. By embracing self-compassion practices, new moms can cultivate a positive and resilient mindset.

8.1.4 Seeking Professional Support When Needed

The transition to motherhood can bring about mental health challenges, and seeking professional support is a proactive step toward prioritizing mental well-being. Explore the role of mental health professionals, including therapists, counselors, and support groups, in providing guidance and support during this transformative period.

Learn about common mental health concerns for new moms, including postpartum depression and anxiety, and the importance of early intervention. Understand the benefits of therapy in providing a safe space for expression, coping strategies, and personalized support. Delve into the role of medication when prescribed by healthcare professionals, recognizing that mental health treatment is a valid and valuable part of maternal care. By seeking professional support when needed, new moms can prioritize their mental well-being and foster a healthy and resilient mindset.

8.2 Time Management Tips for New Moms
Time management becomes a critical skill for new moms juggling the demands of motherhood, household responsibilities, and potentially returning to work. In this section, we'll explore practical time management tips tailored to the unique challenges faced by new moms, helping them navigate their busy schedules while fostering a sense of balance and efficiency.

8.2.1 Embracing a Flexible Routine

The unpredictability of newborns and the demands of motherhood can make rigid schedules challenging to maintain. Explore the concept of embracing a flexible routine that allows for adjustments based on the baby's needs and the mother's energy levels.

Learn about establishing a loose structure for the day, incorporating key activities such as feeding, napping, and self-care. Understand the benefits of adaptability, recognizing that some days may not go as planned, and that's perfectly normal. Delve into the importance of prioritizing essential tasks while being flexible with non-urgent activities. By embracing a flexible routine, new moms can create a sense of order while accommodating the unpredictable nature of caring for a newborn.

8.2.2 Prioritizing Self-Care as Non-Negotiable

Self-care is often viewed as a luxury, but for new moms, it is a non-negotiable aspect of maintaining well-being. Explore strategies for prioritizing self-care by identifying activities that bring joy, relaxation, and a sense of rejuvenation.

Learn about the concept of "micro self-care," incorporating small and manageable self-care practices into daily routines. Understand that self-care is not selfish but essential for maintaining physical and mental health. Delve into the importance of communicating self-care needs with partners, family members, or friends to ensure support. By prioritizing self-care as non-negotiable, new moms can recharge and approach their responsibilities with renewed energy and resilience.

8.2.3 Efficient Time Blocking

Time blocking is a time management technique that can be particularly effective for new moms looking to structure their days. Explore the concept of dividing the day into blocks of time dedicated to specific activities, allowing for focused attention on each task.

Learn about the benefits of efficient time blocking, including increased productivity, reduced decision fatigue, and a sense of accomplishment. Understand the importance of realistic expectations when allocating time to tasks, recognizing that some activities may take longer than anticipated. Delve into the adaptability of time blocking, allowing for adjustments based on the baby's needs and unforeseen circumstances. By implementing efficient time blocking, new moms can make the most of their time and create a sense of order in their daily lives.

8.2.4 Delegating and Sharing Responsibilities

The support of partners, family members, and friends is invaluable for new moms in managing their responsibilities. Explore the concept of delegating tasks and sharing responsibilities, creating a collaborative approach to parenting and household duties.

Learn about effective communication with partners regarding workload distribution and shared responsibilities. Understand that asking for help is a sign of strength, not weakness, and contributes to a healthier family dynamic. Delve into the importance of setting realistic expectations for oneself and others, recognizing that no one can do it all alone. By delegating and sharing responsibilities, new moms can create a support system that enhances efficiency and promotes a balanced lifestyle.

8.2.5 Emphasizing Time for Connection

Amidst the busyness of motherhood, it's crucial to emphasize time for connection—with the baby, partner, and oneself. Explore strategies for carving out intentional moments of connection, fostering meaningful relationships and nurturing emotional well-being.

Learn about the benefits of quality time spent with the baby, including bonding, communication, and fostering a sense of security. Understand the importance of maintaining connection with a partner through shared activities, communication, and mutual support. Delve into the concept of "me time," allowing new moms to engage in activities they enjoy and recharge their emotional reserves. By emphasizing time for connection, new moms can create a balanced and fulfilling life that extends beyond the demands of daily tasks.

8.3 Building a Support System

Building a robust support system is essential for new moms as they navigate the challenges and joys of motherhood. In this section, we'll explore the importance of cultivating a supportive network, including partners, family members, friends, and community resources, to enhance the overall well-being of new moms and create a foundation for a positive motherhood experience.

8.3.1 Recognizing the Role of Partners

Partners play a crucial role in the support system for new moms, contributing to both physical and emotional well-being. Explore the importance of open communication with partners, including discussions about expectations, responsibilities, and shared parenting goals.

Learn about the benefits of mutual support, where partners actively participate in caregiving, household tasks, and emotional reassurance. Understand the significance of partners being attuned to the needs and feelings of new moms, creating a sense of partnership in the journey of parenthood. Delve into the concept of shared decision-making, where partners collaborate on parenting choices and household responsibilities. By recognizing the role of partners in the support system, new moms can strengthen their connection and face the challenges of parenthood as a united team.

8.3.2 Building a Network of Family Support

Family support provides a valuable safety net for new moms, offering assistance, guidance, and emotional reinforcement. Explore strategies for building a network of family support, including grandparents, siblings, and extended family members.

Learn about the benefits of involving family members in caregiving tasks, allowing new moms time for self-care and rest. Understand the importance of open communication with family members, expressing needs, and setting boundaries when necessary. Delve into the concept of family traditions and rituals that contribute to a sense of connection and shared experiences. By building a network of family support, new moms can create a foundation of strength and resilience in the face of the demands of motherhood.

8.3.3 Cultivating Friendships with Fellow Moms
Fellow moms can provide a unique and understanding support system, as they share similar experiences and challenges. Explore the importance of cultivating friendships with fellow moms, whether through prenatal classes, parenting groups, or online communities.

Learn about the benefits of sharing experiences, advice, and resources with other moms who are navigating the same journey. Understand the significance of empathy and non-judgmental support from peers who understand the complexities of motherhood. Delve into the concept of organizing playdates or group activities, fostering social connections for both moms and babies. By cultivating friendships with fellow moms, new moms can build a sense of camaraderie, share insights, and create a supportive community.

8.3.4 Tapping into Community Resources

Community resources provide additional layers of support for new moms, offering a range of services, information, and assistance. Explore the wealth of community resources available, including parenting classes, support groups, and healthcare services.

Learn about the benefits of attending parenting classes, where new moms can gain valuable knowledge, skills, and connections. Understand the importance of seeking out local support groups or online communities that cater to the specific needs and interests of new moms. Delve into the concept of utilizing healthcare services, including postpartum check-ups, lactation consultants, and mental health professionals, to address various aspects of well-being. By tapping into community resources, new moms can access a comprehensive support system that addresses both practical and emotional needs.

8.3.5 Knowing When to Seek Professional Support

While friends and family provide crucial support, there are instances where professional support becomes essential for the well-being of new moms. Explore the signs that indicate the need for professional assistance, including persistent feelings of sadness, anxiety, or difficulty coping with daily tasks.

Learn about the role of healthcare professionals, therapists, and counselors in providing specialized support for mental and emotional well-being. Understand that seeking professional help is a proactive and courageous step toward prioritizing one's health. Delve into the importance of open communication with healthcare providers about mental health concerns, as early intervention can lead to effective support and treatment. By knowing when to seek professional support, new moms can ensure they receive the comprehensive care necessary for a healthy and fulfilling motherhood experience.

CHAPTER 9

Beyond the First Year

9.1 Continuing Your Fitness and Nutrition Journey

The postpartum period extends well beyond the first year, and continuing your fitness and nutrition journey is crucial for sustaining a healthy and fulfilling lifestyle. In this section, we'll explore strategies for maintaining and evolving your fitness and nutrition practices, taking into account the changing dynamics of motherhood.

9.1.1 Evolving Fitness Routines

As your baby grows, so do the opportunities to adapt and evolve your fitness routines. Explore the concept of tailoring your workouts to align with your changing energy levels, time constraints, and personal preferences. Understand the importance of incorporating both cardiovascular exercises and strength training to promote overall health and well-being.

Learn about family-friendly fitness activities that involve your child, such as stroller walks, baby-wearing workouts, and interactive play sessions. Delve into the potential benefits of joining postpartum fitness classes or mom-and-baby exercise groups, fostering a sense of community and motivation. Recognize the significance of consistency in your fitness journey, adjusting your routines as needed to accommodate the demands of motherhood. By evolving your fitness routines, you can seamlessly integrate physical activity into your lifestyle and continue to reap the rewards of an active and healthy life.

9.1.2 Nourishing Your Body for Long-Term Health

Nutrition remains a cornerstone of your well-being beyond the first year of motherhood. Explore strategies for nourishing your body with nutrient-dense foods, emphasizing a balanced and varied diet that meets your evolving nutritional needs.

Learn about adjusting portion sizes and nutrient ratios based on changes in activity levels, lifestyle, and personal health goals. Understand the importance of continuing to prioritize key nutrients such as calcium, iron, and omega-3 fatty acids for your health and the well-being of your growing child. Delve into the concept of meal prepping and planning to maintain a healthy eating routine amid the demands of a busy life. Recognize that your nutritional choices contribute not only to your physical health but also to sustained energy levels and overall vitality as you navigate the ongoing journey of motherhood.

9.1.3 Setting Long-Term Fitness Goals

Setting long-term fitness goals provides a roadmap for your continued journey beyond the first year of motherhood. Explore the concept of establishing realistic and achievable fitness objectives that align with your personal preferences, health aspirations, and time constraints.

Learn about the benefits of setting both short-term and long-term goals, providing milestones to celebrate and adjust as needed. Understand the importance of incorporating a variety of fitness activities to keep your routines engaging and effective. Delve into the potential of working with fitness professionals, such as personal trainers or nutritionists, to create a personalized and sustainable plan. Recognize that your fitness goals are dynamic and can be adjusted to accommodate the ever-changing landscape of motherhood. By setting long-term fitness goals, you empower yourself to cultivate a lasting commitment to your health and well-being.

9.2 Adapting to the Changing Needs of Motherhood

As your child grows, motherhood continues to present new challenges and joys. Adapting to the changing needs of motherhood involves flexible approaches to parenting, self-care, and personal growth. In this section, we'll explore strategies for embracing the evolving dynamics of motherhood and finding balance amid the transitions.

9.2.1 Embracing Milestones and Transitions

Motherhood is marked by a series of milestones and transitions as your child progresses through different developmental stages. Explore the concept of embracing these moments as opportunities for growth, learning, and connection. Understand the importance of adapting your parenting style to align with your child's changing needs, fostering a supportive and responsive relationship.

Learn about the significance of self-reflection and mindfulness in navigating transitions, allowing you to approach changes with a positive mindset. Delve into the potential challenges of balancing your personal and family needs during transitional periods, emphasizing the importance of open communication and flexibility. Recognize that embracing milestones and transitions is not only about your child's growth but also about your evolving role and identity as a mother.

9.2.2 Prioritizing Self-Care Amidst Busy Schedules

As the demands of motherhood evolve, it becomes increasingly crucial to prioritize self-care amidst busy schedules. Explore strategies for integrating self-care practices into your daily routine, recognizing that taking care of yourself is a fundamental aspect of being an effective and fulfilled mother.

Learn about time-efficient self-care activities, such as short mindfulness exercises, quick workouts, or moments of quiet reflection, that can be seamlessly incorporated into your schedule. Understand the importance of setting boundaries and communicating your self-care needs to family members, friends, and partners. Delve into the concept of delegating responsibilities when needed to create time for rejuvenation and relaxation. By prioritizing self-care amidst busy schedules, you ensure that you have the energy and resilience to meet the evolving demands of motherhood.

9.2.3 Fostering Independence in Your Child

As your child grows, fostering independence becomes an integral part of your parenting journey. Explore strategies for encouraging age-appropriate independence in your child, promoting autonomy and confidence.

Learn about providing opportunities for your child to make choices, take on responsibilities, and problem-solve, contributing to their cognitive and emotional development. Understand the importance of balancing guidance and support with the freedom for your child to explore and learn from their experiences. Delve into the potential challenges of letting go as a parent and allowing your child to navigate certain situations independently. Recognize that fostering independence in your child not only benefits their growth but also allows you the space to attend to your own needs and interests.

9.2.4 Navigating Work-Life Integration

For mothers who have returned to work, navigating work-life integration is an ongoing process that requires adaptability and effective time management. Explore strategies for balancing professional responsibilities with family life, recognizing that the integration of these aspects is dynamic and subject to change.

Learn about the benefits of open communication with employers regarding flexible work arrangements, understanding that a supportive work environment contributes to a healthy work-life balance. Understand the importance of setting realistic expectations for both work and home life, acknowledging that perfection is not attainable. Delve into the potential challenges of managing guilt or pressure associated with divided attention between work and family, emphasizing the importance of self-compassion. Recognize that navigating work-life integration is a continuous journey, and adjustments may be needed as your child grows and your professional and personal priorities evolve.

9.3 Celebrating Your Ongoing Success

Celebrating your ongoing success as a mother involves recognizing and appreciating the milestones, personal growth, and resilience you've demonstrated throughout the journey of motherhood. In this section, we'll explore the importance of acknowledging your achievements, embracing self-reflection, and finding joy in the ongoing success of your parenting experience.

9.3.1 Reflecting on Personal Growth

Motherhood is a transformative journey that fosters personal growth and self-discovery. Take the time to reflect on the ways in which you have evolved as an individual since becoming a mother.

Explore the personal strengths and qualities you've developed, such as patience, resilience, and adaptability. Understand the impact of your experiences on your perspectives, values, and priorities. Delve into the potential challenges you've overcome and the lessons you've learned along the way. By reflecting on your personal growth, you can gain a deeper understanding of yourself and celebrate the ongoing evolution that comes with the responsibilities of motherhood.

9.3.2 Acknowledging Parenting Milestones

Parenting is a journey marked by numerous milestones, both big and small. Acknowledge and celebrate these milestones as a testament to your dedication, love, and commitment to your child's well-being.

Learn about the significance of recognizing developmental milestones in your child, such as their first steps, first words, and academic achievements. Understand the emotional impact of these moments on your parenting journey and the sense of pride they evoke. Delve into the concept of creating meaningful traditions or rituals to commemorate these milestones, fostering a sense of joy and connection within the family. By acknowledging parenting milestones, you can savor the unique moments that contribute to the tapestry of your ongoing success as a mother.

9.3.3 Finding Joy in Everyday Moments

Amidst the challenges and busyness of motherhood, finding joy in everyday moments is essential for maintaining a positive outlook and emotional well-being. Explore strategies for cultivating mindfulness and appreciating the simple pleasures that occur in your daily life.

Learn about the benefits of being present in the moment, whether it's sharing a laughter-filled meal with your family, witnessing your child's curiosity, or enjoying quiet moments of reflection. Understand the role of gratitude in fostering a positive mindset, acknowledging the blessings and positive aspects of your life. Delve into the potential challenges of balancing responsibilities and finding time for personal enjoyment, emphasizing the importance of creating space for joy in your routine. By finding joy in everyday moments, you can infuse your parenting journey with positivity and create a lasting sense of fulfillment.

9.3.4 Celebrating Self-Care Achievements

Self-care achievements are worth celebrating as they contribute to your overall well-being and resilience as a mother. Explore the concept of acknowledging and commemorating the efforts you invest in your self-care practices.

Learn about setting personal self-care goals and milestones, whether it's maintaining a consistent fitness routine, prioritizing mental health, or cultivating a hobby. Understand the importance of recognizing and applauding your achievements, no matter how small they may seem. Delve into the potential challenges of balancing self-care with other responsibilities and the societal expectations placed on mothers. Recognize that celebrating self-care achievements is an affirmation of your commitment to your own health and happiness.

9.3.5 Building a Supportive Community

The community you surround yourself with plays a significant role in your ongoing success as a mother. Explore the importance of building and maintaining a supportive community that uplifts, encourages, and celebrates your journey.

Learn about the benefits of connecting with other mothers who share similar experiences and challenges. Understand the impact of positive relationships with family, friends, and mentors who provide emotional support and practical assistance. Delve into the concept of reciprocal support, where you contribute to the well-being of others in your community. Recognize that building a supportive community enhances your resilience, provides a sense of belonging, and amplifies the celebration of your ongoing success as a mother.

CONCLUSION

In the comprehensive guide to exercise for first-time moms and the accompanying cookbook, the journey of motherhood unfolds with wisdom and practicality. From embracing fitness during pregnancy to postpartum recovery, the guide provides invaluable insights. Complemented by the nutritious delights of the cookbook, it's a holistic resource for first-time moms. Beyond the initial stages, it encourages an enduring commitment to fitness, adapting to evolving needs. The conclusion celebrates the resilience of mothers, emphasizing personal growth, acknowledging milestones, finding joy, and fostering a supportive community. Together, the guide and cookbook serve as empowering companions on the remarkable journey of motherhood.